TRADITIONAL
REMEDIES

TRADITIONAL REMEDIES

Linda Gray

EBURY
PRESS

615 888 .

Originally published in Great Britain in 1994
This edition published by Ebury Publishing in 2007

1 3 5 7 9 10 8 6 4 2

Text © Linda Gray 1994
Cover design by Estuary English

Ebury Publishing
Random House, 20 Vauxhall Bridge Road, London SW1V 2SA

Random House Australia (Pty) Limited
20 Alfred Street, Milsons Point, Sydney, New South Wales 2061, Australia

Random House New Zealand Limited
18 Poland Road, Glenfield, Auckland 10, New Zealand

Random House South Africa (Pty) Limited
Isle of Houghton, Corner Boundary Road & Carse O'Gowrie, Houghton, 2198, South Africa

Random House Publishers India Private Limited
301 World Trade Tower, Hotel Intercontinental Grand Complex, Barakhamba Lane,
New Delhi 110 001, India

The Random House Group Limited Reg. No. 954009
www.randomhouse.co.uk

A CIP catalogue record for this book is available from the British Library.

ISBN: 0091917859
ISBN-13: 9780091917852

Papers used by Ebury Press are natural, recyclable products made from
wood grown in sustainable forests.

Printed and bound in China by Leo Paper Products

Contents

Introduction

LONG BEFORE the discovery of modern medicines, families used remedies based on plants to treat everyday illness. Instructions were passed down through the generations, until fast-acting antibiotics and analgesics became available and folk medicine gradually fell into disuse. Now there's a tremendous revival of interest in these home remedies. Not only are they often gentler than manufactured drugs, but many of them are now known to be effective too. It has been discovered that meadowsweet and willow bark, used by families 150 years ago to soothe pain and relieve fever, contain salicin – aspirin. Today, plants are a source of many powerful drugs for those modern plagues, heart disease and cancer.

Like other drugs, plants can harm as well as heal, which is why this book concentrates on remedies that are safe for all the family. Even so, none should be taken in pregnancy or for major illnesses, combined with other medicines, or given to babies under one, without medical advice. As a rule, if your symptoms are new for you, or continue for more than a week, you should see your GP. Many of the remedies recommended in this book are in the form of herbal teas, and you can make them up to suit your own taste. It's better to take a weak infusion regularly than an unpalatably strong one occasionally. Keep all medicines, including essential oils, out of the reach of children.

Traditional medicine is based on natural plants rather than isolated chemicals, often for good reason. Dandelions, for example, can help prevent water retention. But unlike other diuretics, which can deplete the body's potassium supplies, dandelions contain stores of this valuable mineral to make sure the correct balance is maintained. This holistic or 'whole body' approach means that many old-fashioned remedies need time to act. Teas, washes and compresses are best incorporated into your everyday routine, especially if you want to treat chronic conditions or stress. Try them. They're safe, effective, simple to use, and a living link with the past.

CHAPTER ONE

Aches & Pains

*T*here's a wonderful variety of traditional remedies for rheumatism — possibly a reflection of the problems people faced when living in damp or unheated houses. Today, central heating has improved living conditions inside, but the climate hasn't changed and arthritic aches and pains are as much a problem as ever. Many people who are affected instinctively know when it's going to rain and find they feel better when the weather is dry. Wearing a copper bracelet is one folk remedy that's said to help; you can buy special bangles from pharmacists. If you're still plagued by joint pains, try the following remedies.

Meadowsweet Compress

MEADOWSWEET IS nature's pain reliever, and soothes
aching joints. It grows wild or in the garden and is
available dried from herbalists. Meadowsweet is one of
the original sources of aspirin, an anti-inflammatory
drug that fights both pain and swelling. As many people
with arthritis know, aspirin and similar drugs can also
wreak havoc with the digestive tract but unlike the
extracted drug, meadowsweet contains ingredients that
protect the stomach.

To make a compress, pour $\frac{1}{2}$ pint (275 ml) of freshly
boiled (not boiling) water over $1\frac{1}{2}$ oz (40 g) of fresh
meadowsweet leaves and flowers or $\frac{1}{2}$ oz (15 g) of dried.
Cover and leave for 10 minutes. When it has cooled
sufficiently to be comfortable to the touch, soak a pad of
clean cotton or cotton wool in the liquid, squeeze out the
excess and hold the pad against the skin until it dries or
cools. Repeat as necessary, using the warm liquid.

Honey and Cider Vinegar

MANY PEOPLE swear by this sweet and sour remedy for arthritis, believing that it clears toxins from the system.

Add 1 teaspoon of runny honey and 1 teaspoon of apple cider vinegar to a cup of hot water and drink it daily.

❖

Celery Tea

CELERY STIMULATES the kidneys and helps flush out the system, which can help arthritis and gout. The seeds are more potent than the plant, but gather them fresh or buy them from herbalists. Avoid seeds from garden centres, as they may have been chemically treated to make them pest-resistant.

Add 1 heaped teaspoon of celery seeds to a mug of boiling water and infuse for 10 minutes, then strain. Take 3 times a day.

Herbal Baths

A HERBAL bath can be soothing or stimulating, depending on the plants you choose. You can make a bath bag with dried herbs sewn into a square of muslin, or opt for the stronger pure essential oils that aromatherapists use. Keep them firmly stoppered in glass bottles in a cool dark place.

To soak away aches and pains, take equal parts of essential oil of rosemary, thyme and horse chestnut and mix together. Shake well and add a few drops to your bath water.

❖

Garlic Cloves

GARLIC IS a home remedy for earache and guaranteed, so country lore has it, to draw the pain if the ear is inflamed.

Peel a clove of garlic and cut it if necessary, so that it fits just inside the ear. Wrap it in a piece of gauze or fine cotton, and replace every few hours.

Cowslip Pain Relief

THE COWSLIP is doubly useful. Like meadowsweet, the root has similar properties to aspirin, while the flowers have a sedative effect. As the cowslip is also good for coughs and colds, the whole plant has a place in relieving aches and pains. Picking wild flowers is no longer acceptable, but why not grow them in your garden or windowbox? Some people are sensitive to the plant, so try the compress first, rather than the tea, to test for allergy.

Divide the cowslips into roots and flowers. Place 3 oz (75 g) of root in a pan and cover with 1 pint (550 ml) of cold water. Bring to the boil and simmer for 1 hour, then strain into a jug. When the liquid has cooled sufficiently to be comfortable to the touch, wring out a cotton cloth in it and apply to the aching joint.

Take 1 1/2 oz (40 g) of cowslip flowers, add 1/2 pint (275 ml) of freshly boiled water and infuse for 10 minutes. Soak a cotton pad in the liquid, wring out, and apply to the face to relieve neuralgia. This also makes a pleasant tea, good for insomnia.

Rosemary Oil Massage

A ROSEMARY oil massage helps combat stiffness and lifts the spirits too. Try a few drops in the bath or add to the power of touch, in a soothing massage.

Blend 5 drops of essential oil of rosemary with 1 tablespoon of a neutral carrier oil (almond is best). Massage into the skin to restore movement and relieve pain.

❖

Wintergreen and Cider Vinegar Rheumatism Rub

THIS COMBINES two favourites for relieving rheumatism – oil of wintergreen to improve circulation and cider vinegar to ease the pain. Some people are sensitive to wintergreen oil, so test a little of the mixture first and leave for 24 hours to make sure that it doesn't irritate your skin.

Mix $\frac{1}{2}$ teaspoon of wintergreen oil with $\frac{1}{2}$ pint (275 ml) of cider vinegar. Soak a cotton pad in the mixture, wring out and hold against the affected area.

Headaches

IT'S NORMAL to have headaches: 98 per cent of people do. That doesn't make them any easier to bear, particularly if you suffer from the incapacitating misery of migraine, where blurred vision and nausea add to the distress. Fortunately there's help at hand in the form of traditional remedies, some of which have been used for three centuries and are now winning scientific acceptance.

Headache Tea

THIS RECIPE is a traditional family favourite. Cinnamon and ginger offset the side effects of a sick headache.

Pour 1 cup of water and $1/2$ glass of milk into a small saucepan. Add a 1 inch (2.5 cm) piece of peeled fresh ginger root, a large stick of cinnamon and 1 teaspoon of strong tea leaves and bring to the boil. Leave it to brew over a low heat for 5 minutes, then strain and add sugar to taste.

Feverfew Leaves

FEVERFEW IS a herb with feathery leaves and pretty, daisy-like flowers. It grows freely in many gardens all year round. Used since the 18th century to prevent migraine, it's now accepted by the British Migraine Association and is under scientific scrutiny. It seems to work by regulating the flow of blood to the brain – certainly 70 per cent of people in trials reported that they felt better for taking it.

Eat 2 or 3 fresh leaves daily, chopped in a sandwich to disguise the bitter taste; dried leaves can be eaten in the same way. Feverfew sometimes causes mouth ulcers or itchy skin; if this happens to you, try one of the other remedies in this chapter instead.

Lavender Rub

LAVENDER IS antiseptic, relaxing and deliciously scented
– just what's needed when a headache strikes.

Take the pure essential oil aromatherapists use and add 5
drops to 1 tablespoon of almond oil. Massage it slowly into
your temples and the nape of your neck. After the
massage, sit down and put your head between your knees.
Massage your scalp gently and relax.

❖

Headache Cushion

A HEADACHE cushion is filled with soothing herbs.
Slip it under your pillow for sound sleep and
sweeter dreams.

Make up a bag from a square of cotton lawn and fill it
with dried lavender, marjoram, rose leaves and petals,
wood betony and a scattering of crushed cloves.

Ginger Poultice

A GINGER poultice can help relieve that pounding feeling in your head. Unlike a compress, which is a pad dipped in a liquid or lotion then pressed on the affected area, a poultice applies the active ingredients directly to the skin. It can be kept in place by a lint bandage if necessary.

Add a little water to 1 tablespoon of powdered ginger and heat gently in a small saucepan until it forms a paste. Test to make sure it won't burn your skin, then spread the warm paste over your forehead, taking care that none of it trickles into your eyes. Lie down in a quiet, darkened room, leaving the poultice in place until it has cooled.

Quick Tips

A jacket potato, eaten plain, helps alleviate the nausea of migraine.

Half a raw onion held against a bruise encourages it to disappear.

Dab one drop of *oil of cloves* on an aching tooth.

Peeled and washed *raw potato* can restore moisture to small burns and ease the pain.

Warmed olive oil loosens ear wax – put a little in the ear and keep in place with cotton wool.

Honey may help to heal wounds.

Three juniper berries eaten daily may ward off rheumatism.

Place raw steak on a black eye.

Warm cabbage leaves are good for sprains – secure with a crepe bandage.

Warmed almond oil soothes earache – put a little in the ear and keep in place with cotton wool.

A rosemary oil scalp rub lifts headaches.

CHAPTER TWO

Coughs, Colds & Fevers

*T*here are probably more traditional remedies for these ailments than for any other category of illness — and no wonder when there are about 200 viruses responsible for the sneezing, wheezing and general discomfort caused by the common cold. Now that doctors are trying to limit the use of antibiotics (which in any case can't help if you have a viral infection) it's a good time to look again at some of the tried and tested ways in which families have relieved the symptoms of both colds and flu.

Four Thieves' Vinegar

THIS IS a splendid traditional favourite for preventing infection. It's based on the legend of four thieves, arrested for looting during a plague, who were granted their freedom in exchange for disclosing the recipe that protected them from disease. It can be taken internally, diluted and used as a sick-room cleanser, or added to a bath.

Blend together 2 teaspoons of crushed garlic with 2 teaspoons of each of the following dried herbs: lavender, rosemary, sage and mint. (The original recipe also includes mugwort and rue, but these are very powerful herbs and you should seek the advice of a qualified herbalist before using them.) Put the herbs into a screw-top jar and cover with 1 pint (550 ml) of cider vinegar. Leave in a warm place for 2 weeks, then strain and decant into a clean bottle. Take 2 teaspoons 3 times a day.

Linseed Tea

LINSEED TEA is 'very good for a cold or sore throat', according to one *Good Housekeeping* reader whose family used it regularly. Linseed is derived from flax and was commonly used in poultices for burns and for a range of internal complaints. It is also a common remedy for constipation. Here, spices and flavourings are added to make it more palatable.

Rinse 2 oz (50 g) of linseed in a sieve and put it in a saucepan with 1³/₄ pints (1 litre) of cold water, 4 strips of lemon rind, 4 cloves and 1 teaspoon of powdered cinnamon. Bring the mixture gently to the boil and simmer for 1 hour. Add the juice of 1 lemon and sugar to taste, stir, and strain into a jug. Cover, cool, and keep refrigerated, heating as much as you require at a time.

Honey and Lemon Cough Linctus

THESE TWO traditional cold remedies are given a kick
by a third – whisky – so this is for adults only. It
has certainly stood the test of time. This recipe
was handed down to Mrs Joyce Slater by
her grandmother, born in 1867.

Whisk 1 tablespoon each of clear honey, whisky, lemon
juice and glycerine in 4 tablespoons of warm water. Take
1 tablespoon, 3 times a day.

❖

Mustard Plaster

A MUSTARD plaster sounds straight out of Dickens, but
it's comforting, warm, and bound to help you feel better
if your chest is tight.

Mix 1 part of mustard powder with 4 parts of flour and
add sufficient water to work to a thick paste. Rub a little
warmed olive oil over the chest and then apply the
mustard paste, keeping it in place with strips of clean
cotton (an old sheet will do). Apply to your back too, if
you like.

Fragrant Catarrh Cure

THIS COMBINATION of sweetly scented antibacterial and stimulant herbs can be used as a chest rub (diluted in a neutral oil such as almond or olive) or inhaled, to make breathing easier. Why not try both?

Mix 1 drop each of essential oils of chamomile, lavender, eucalyptus and peppermint in 2 tablespoons of carrier oil for a chest rub. If you'd rather inhale them, add the same number of drops to a basin of boiling water. Cover both your head and the basin with a towel and breathe in deeply.

❖

Red Sage Gargle

RED SAGE is an excellent remedy for a sore throat and more potent than its kitchen garden cousin.

Add 1 heaped teaspoon of dried red sage to 1 mug of boiling water and leave to stand for 10 minutes. Strain, then add 1 teaspoon of cider vinegar. The infusion can also be sipped as a tea, but may be too strong for some tastes.

Garlic and Ginger Toddy

GARLIC AND ginger combine in this invigorating toddy that's hot in more ways than one! Garlic is great for colds; in fact, you're advised to chew several cloves of fresh garlic a day to fend off infection – or repel those likely to pass it on to you. Ginger is warming and can help combat the queasy feeling that so often comes with blocked sinuses or the stubborn cough it's designed to shift.

Peel 4 cloves of garlic and 1 inch (2.5 cm) of fresh ginger root and put them in a saucepan with 1 pint (550 ml) of cold water. Add 6 mint leaves and 10 black peppercorns, bring to the boil and simmer for half an hour. Strain into a jug and drink 1 cup every 3 hours. It's particularly effective taken piping hot.

Raspberry Vinegar

VINEGARS ARE a traditional way of preserving all the goodness of fruit, either for cooking or, as here, for the medicine chest. Raspberry vinegar is soothing for sore throats.

Put $^1/_2$ lb (250 g) of raspberries into a large, wide-necked jar and cover with $^3/_4$ pint (415 ml) of cider vinegar. Seal and leave for 3 weeks. Strain thoroughly, decant into a clean bottle and use as a gargle, or sip a spoonful at a time, as a cough medicine.

❖

Salt Water Snifter

FOR A traditional decongestant, try this salt water snifter.

Add $^1/_4$ teaspoon of table salt to $^1/_2$ glass of water and transfer to a small pan. Bring to the boil then leave to cool. Sniff 2 to 3 drops up each nostril to clear a blocked nose.

Blackcurrant Cordial

BLACKCURRANT CORDIAL is a very pleasant way of warding off colds and making sniffles and sore throats more bearable. The berries are an excellent source of vitamin C; harvest and freeze them during the summer so that you have enough to see you through the winter.

Put 1 lb (500 g) of prepared blackcurrants in a heavy-based saucepan with 1 teaspoon each of ground cloves, nutmeg and cinnamon. Add water to cover, bring to the boil and simmer until soft. Sieve to remove the skins, then strain and sweeten to taste with honey. Drink a sherry glassful as needed.

Herbal Chest Rub

THIS CONTAINS antibacterial lavender and tea tree oils to fight infection.

Dilute 2 drops of lavender oil and 1 drop of tea tree oil in 1 tablespoon of almond oil. Rub into your chest, back, hands and feet morning and night.

Oil of Eucalyptus

THE PUNGENT aroma of oil of eucalyptus (traditionally known as the fever tree) gets through however stuffy your nose. Scatter a few drops on a handkerchief and breathe in the vapours, or sprinkle a little on your pillow at night; add five drops to one tablespoon of olive or almond oil to massage into your chest; gargle with a few drops in a glass of warm water, or inhale, as follows, to relieve a heavy cold.

Add 4 drops of eucalyptus oil to a small bowl of freshly boiled water, cover both your head and the bowl with a towel and breathe in the steam as deeply as you can for several minutes. If you prefer, you can also use a facial sauna or special inhaling cup instead, available from pharmacists.

Beef Tea

THIS IS an old favourite that's just as beneficial today as it was in Victorian times. It can help rebuild your strength if you're feeling run down or recovering from a bout of flu, especially if you have a tendency to anaemia. The long cooking time makes it easy to digest.

Cut away the fat from ½ lb (250 g) of rump steak, chop the steak roughly and put it into a food processor for a few seconds until finely shredded. Transfer it to a pudding bowl and add ½ pint (275 ml) of water and a little fresh or dried parsley, thyme, rosemary and marjoram. Cover with a pudding cloth and leave for an hour or so before placing it in a saucepan containing enough water to come halfway up the side of the bowl. Cover the pan with a lid, bring the water to the boil and simmer gently for 3 hours, topping up with water as necessary. Sieve to remove the fibres, then skim. Leave until cold, remove the fat and heat to serve. Add salt to taste.

Onion

ONION IS an excellent soother for sore throats. Serve it savoury or sweet, as you prefer. Here are two traditional recipes.

1) Boil a whole onion until tender and eat with plenty of butter and seasoning.
2) Finely chop a raw onion, place in a dish and cover generously with thin honey. Leave for 24 hours, then remove the onion. Take 2 teaspoons of the honey twice daily until better.

❖

Tonic Rub

A TONIC rub made from natural eucalyptus and tea tree oils is pleasant to use and helps boost immunity. Use it whenever you are feeling particularly tired and run down.

Take 2 drops each of eucalyptus and tea tree oil and dilute in 2 tablespoons of a neutral carrier oil. Rub it into your hands, feet and glands to improve immunity.

White Willow Fever Tea

WHITE WILLOW fever tea was granny's answer to today's hot lemon cold remedies. Like meadowsweet, white willow contains similar ingredients to aspirin, and so can reduce pain and fever. Pick fresh leaves, which have a very mild effect, or, for more relief, try capsules of powdered bark, available from herbalists.

Take 2 oz (50 g) of fresh white willow leaves and cover with 1 pint (550 ml) of boiling water. Leave to stand for 10 minutes, then strain. Sweeten to taste and drink.

Spice Oils

INHALING SPICE oils with a sedative effect can soothe an irritating cough and help you to a good night's sleep.

Add 2 drops each of frankincense and sandalwood oils to a basin of freshly boiled water. Put a towel over both your head and the basin and breathe in deeply.

Elderberry Tonic

AN ELDERBERRY tonic was frequently recommended in the past to shift coughs. Elderberries and elderflowers were also popular ingredients in homemade wines, which must have made a cold far easier to bear. This recipe contains no alcohol but it does have plenty of vitamin C to help fight a cold.

Put 4 oz (125 g) of elderberries in a pan with 6 cloves and add enough cold water to cover. Bring to the boil then reduce the heat, cover, and simmer until soft. Sieve the berries or put them through a blender. Add sugar to taste, plus a sprig of fresh thyme if you have a particularly troublesome cough. Take a sherryglassful at regular intervals.

Quick Tips

Apply a *block of salt in a hot cloth* to your face to draw sinus pains.

Kaolin ointment smeared round the neck is good for sore throats.

Gargle with *salt water* – a teaspoon of salt in a glass of water – twice daily to relieve a sore throat.

Take half a teaspoon of *turmeric powder in a glass of hot milk* for colds.

Spray *lemon juice* on the back of a sore throat.

Chew *honeycomb* to clear sinusitis.

Inhale *Friar's Balsam* (tincture of benzoin) for a blocked-up nose.

A sprig of rosemary in red wine fights infection.

Cold baths are said to boost immunity!

CHAPTER THREE

Skin

*I*n the days before mass-produced skincare products, healing ointments and washes were often made up in the kitchen, where everyday ingredients like oatmeal and glycerine were to hand. Combined with herbs and flowers from the garden, they were used to treat all kinds of ailments, from sores and chapped hands to acne and eczema – a gentle, natural alternative to chemical skin treatments.

Marigold Rinse

MARIGOLD RINSE is invaluable for the treatment of all kinds of skin conditions. Pot marigold has been cultivated for centuries for its soothing antiseptic and antifungal action; Henry VII even recommended using it as a cure for the plague. Today, it is well worth trying this refreshing rinse for healing minor wounds, soothing ezcema and sore skin, and treating complaints like roundworm and athlete's foot.

Put 4 oz (125 g) of fresh marigold heads or 2 oz (50 g) of dried in a large jug and cover with 1 pint (550 ml) of freshly boiled water. Leave until pleasantly cool to the touch, then strain into a basin. Apply to the affected area with clean cotton or cotton wool. Add an equal quantity of cider vinegar to the rinse if you want to reduce inflammation.

Lavender Wash

LAVENDER IS wonderful for first aid because it's antiseptic and soothes bites and small burns. You can use it for inflammatory skin conditions too. A lavender wash can help keep spots at bay.

Cover 4 oz (125 g) of fresh lavender flowers or 2 oz (50 g) of dried with 1 pint (550 ml) of freshly boiled water and leave to cool. Rinse your face with it night and morning. Reinforce its action by applying neat essential oil of lavender to any particularly troublesome spots.

Lavender Vinegar

LAVENDER VINEGAR is more astringent than a lavender wash, and it's a traditional way to combat acne. Diluted with water, it makes a refreshing skin tonic.

Put 1 cup of freshly picked lavender flowers into a screw-top jar and cover with white vinegar. Store in a cool, dark place for a week, shaking once a day, then strain and pour into a clean jar or bottle.

Oatmeal

OATMEAL IS traditionally used to soften dry skin. You can simply scatter it in the bath (wonderful to relieve itching), rub it into your hands and face, or tie a cup of oats, half a cup of bran and two cups of soap powder in a pudding cloth and simmer to make a soap substitute. Alternatively, why not make an oatmeal poultice to help heal chapped skin?

Mix a handful of oatmeal to a paste with a little warm water. Apply directly to the skin and bind it with gauze or cotton strips to keep the oatmeal in place. Leave until cool, or for longer if liked.

Cabbage Lotion

CABBAGE – THE medicine of the poor – has a gently anti-inflammatory action that can help subdue spots.

Pulp $^1/_2$ 1b (250 g) of cabbage leaves, stripped of their stalks and woody ribs, in a food processor, then mix with $^1/_2$ pint (275 ml) of distilled witch hazel. Add $^1/_2$ teaspoon of lemon juice and stir well. Apply twice a day.

Cucumber Lotion

CUCUMBER HAS a mild bleaching action, much appreciated in Victorian times for its ability to fade freckles. No one considers freckles unsightly now, but you can try it to fade blemishes and age spots.

Peel half a cucumber and liquidize to obtain the juice. Add an equal amount of glycerine and rosewater and stir well. Use as a hand lotion or facial wash.

❖

Rosewater Wash

ROSEWATER IS a traditional skin freshener. The rosewater you buy from pharmacists is what's left when essential oil of rose – one of the most expensive constituents of scent – is distilled. You can also try using the petals of wild roses to make a wash.

Take 3 oz (75 g) of fresh rose petals or 1 ¹/₂ oz (40 g) of dried and pour over 1 pint (550 ml) of freshly boiled water. Leave to cool then strain. Add a little glycerine if your skin is dry, or distilled witch hazel if it's oily.

Wheatgerm Oil

THIS WAS grandmother's answer to anti-ageing creams and quite rightly, because it contains vitamin E. Vitamin E is an important anti-oxidant which attacks the free radicals responsible for cell damage, causing wrinkles, among other things. It's also useful for treating inflammation and wounds, because it helps heal damaged skin. Try massaging a teaspoon of wheatgerm oil into the complexion at bedtime, then rinse with rosewater to remove surface stickiness. Alternatively, add marigold heads to make this healing lotion.

Take 4 tablespoons of fresh marigold heads or 2 tablespoons of dried and put in a jar with 8 tablespoons of wheatgerm oil. Cover and leave to macerate for 3 days, shaking daily, before straining into a clean bottle.

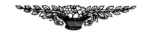

Sugar-and-Soap Poultice

'THIS WAS my grandmother's standby for drawing
out splinters or for bringing spots to a head. I
find it invaluable,' says *Good Housekeeping*
reader Elaine Burrows.

Mash together equal quantities of sugar and soap to make
a poultice. Dab on the spot or splinter, cover with a
plaster and leave overnight. In the morning, remove the
poultice and wash the area. Gently ease the splinter out
or remove the head of the spot with a clean tissue or
comedone spoon, available from pharmacies.

Strawberry Sunburn Soother

STRAWBERRIES ARE a time-honoured way of
soothing sunburn, and luckily the two are in season
at around the same time. Avoid this remedy if you are
allergic to strawberries.

Mash $1/2$ lb (250 g) of overripe strawberries then stir in
$1/2$ pot of plain live yoghurt. Spread the mixture over the
skin to cool it.

Oranges

EATING ORANGES is good for the skin, because they're packed with the anti-oxidant vitamins that help prevent cell damage. They're also useful applied externally too, especially if you use neroli oil, an essential oil distilled from orange blossom and named after the princess who discovered it. She used it to scent her gloves; you can try it to soften your hands.

For a healing skin cream, add 2 drops of neroli oil to 1 teaspoon of bland cream designed for dry skins, such as aqueous cream, available from pharmacies. Mix well and use to relieve soreness or irritation.

Carrot Ointment

CARROT OINTMENT can bring welcome relief to chapped and irritated skin. Carrots have been valued for their soothing, moisturizing properties for years, but it has only recently been discovered that their effectiveness is probably due to the anti-oxidant, vitamin A.

Melt a large jar of white petroleum jelly in a basin placed over a saucepan of hot water. Add 2 tablespoons of grated carrot and simmer gently for 2 hours. While still hot, strain through a muslin cloth into clean pots and allow to cool.

❖

Chickweed Oil

CHICKWEED IS said to spring up wherever hens were kept, and it is certainly a pest in many gardens. Turn it to good account by making it into an oil to ease the irritation caused by sore skin and dermatitis.

Pour $^1/_2$ pint (275 ml) of sunflower oil into a basin set over a pan of hot water and add $^3/_4$ lb (375 g) of freshly gathered chickweed. Simmer gently for 2 hours, topping up the water as necessary, then strain while still warm into a clean bottle. Add 1 tablespoon to the water for a soothing bath.

Quick Tips

Apply slices of *fresh pineapple* to warts.

Distilled witch hazel is good for acne.

Cold weak tea makes a soothing wash for sunburn.

Rub *basil leaves* on stings.

Half a teaspoon of *sea salt* mixed with two tablespoons of *oil* makes a stimulating scrub for tired skin.

White petroleum jelly makes a superb night cream.

Marshmallow root, pounded and simmered, soothes delicate skin.

Hold *geranium leaves* against oily skin to tone it.

Castor oil may fade liver spots.

A little *glycerine* mixed with a pinch of *turmeric powder* can help for mouth ulcers.

A teaspoon of *sugar* mixed with a tablespoon of *olive oil* softens the hands.

CHAPTER FOUR

Hair

*F*rom chamomile and rosemary to beer and vinegar, the kitchen garden and the pantry have always provided the ingredients for the shampoos and rinses needed for a healthy head of hair. You probably pay handsomely for these when they appear in commercial products, so why not try them in their natural state, and reap the full benefit?

A good diet is the most important factor for strong, lustrous hair: make sure you eat lots of green salad and include plenty of fresh herbs, particularly watercress and dill. Then pamper yourself with the time-tested recipes in this chapter to give your hair extra shine.

Herbal Rinse

A HERBAL rinse is the traditional way to add shine and to
bring out the colour of every hair type. Traditional
favourites are chamomile for fair hair, pot marigold for
red or chestnut hair, marjoram or rosemary for dark
hair, elderflower or marshmallow for dry hair and
mint or lavender for greasy hair.

Make a herbal tea, using 1 oz (25 g) of dried herbs or
2 oz (50 g) of fresh, to 1 pint (550 ml) of freshly boiled
water. Allow to stand for 15 minutes, then strain twice
through coffee filter paper. Shampoo and rinse your hair
as normal, before rinsing with the herbal rinse of your
choice.

❖

Scalp Massage

A SCALP massage is a traditional Indian way to unwind.
It relieves knots of tension in your head and neck and
encourages the flow of blood to your brain to perk you
up. Use a few drops of essential oil in a tablespoon of
carrier oil to suit the condition of your hair and your

mood – lavender for greasy hair and to help you relax, rosemary to invigorate, geranium to soothe and moisturize dry hair.

Rub a little of the blended oil of your choice into your hands. Make a fist with each hand and then extend your fingers slightly, keeping them braced. Starting at the nape of your neck, massage your scalp in sections, working methodically round your head.

❖

Egg Conditioner

EGGS WERE what grandmother used to make her hair shine. They're best used as a pre-wash conditioner, to cosset dull and damaged hair.

Dampen your hair and then beat a large egg until it is foamy. Massage into the hair and cover with a shower cap. Leave for 20–30 minutes, then rinse and shampoo as normal.

Warm Oil Remedy

THIS HAIR rescue recipe is warm and sticky but does wonders for dry, damaged hair and split ends. It relies on hot oil, lots of warm towels, and plenty of time. Olive oil suits all hair types, but you can try sunflower oil for fair hair and walnut oil for dark.

Place 2 tablespoons of oil (see above) in an egg cup and warm it by standing the egg cup in a cup or basin of hot water. Work the oil into the hair and scalp and comb through with a wide-toothed comb. Wring out a hand-towel in hot water, wrap it round your head and cover with cling film. When it cools, repeat with another towel – you may need three altogether. After 40–60 minutes, wash your hair with a mild shampoo, using two applications, and rinse until your hair is squeaky clean.

Quick Tips

Beer adds body to fine, flyaway hair – use in the final rinse.

Add a teaspoonful of *vinegar* to the final rinse to make dark hair shine.

Powdered *orris root*, available from herbalists, makes an excellent dry shampoo.

Lavender water, applied with a soft cloth, removes excess oil from greasy hair.

Drink *sage tea* for thick and healthy hair.

Rub *onions* into the roots to strengthen fragile hair.

Add *lemon juice* to the final rinse for oily hair.

CHAPTER FIVE

Eyes

*I*t's well known that people are attracted to faces with wide eyes — which is one reason why Victorian ladies resorted to belladonna, or deadly nightshade, to dilate their pupils. That's not recommended, because belladonna is a poison, but there are many safe and simple traditional ways to soothe sore eyes that are well worth copying today. A number of herbs, such as eyebright, chamomile and elderflower, have been used for centuries to make refreshing lotions and eyebaths which are invaluable for reducing puffiness and relieving eyestrain. All the preparations in this chapter should be applied fresh.

Eyebright

EYEBRIGHT, OR euphrasia, has been valued throughout Europe for centuries for its reputation for sharpening sight and treating infection. Culpeper wrote about it in his famous *Herbal*, adding that it can improve memory as well as the eyesight. Interested? It is easy to grow, and you can take it as a tea as well as using it to soothe your eyes, but unless you want to drink it make up only a small quantity at a time. Eyes are delicate, so any eyewash should be stored in the fridge and kept for a maximum of two days.

Put 1 tablespoon of chopped fresh eyebright leaves, stems and flowers in a saucepan and cover with a mug of cold water. Bring to the boil and simmer for 10 minutes, then strain twice through coffee filter paper. Leave to cool, then refrigerate. To bathe your eyes, use a sterilized eyebath and apply the mixture to each eye, rinsing the eyebath out after each treatment so you don't transfer any infection.

Golden Seal

GOLDEN SEAL is a traditional antiseptic that
can be combined with eyebright or used alone.
It is available from herbalists.

Simmer $^1/_2$ teaspoon of powdered root (available from
herbalists) in 1 mug of water for 10 minutes. Strain twice
through filter paper and dilute with an equal amount of
cool boiled water. Apply as for eyebright.

Chamomile and Elderflower

THESE TWO soothing herbs make a healing mix for
bathing the eyes.

Take 1 tablespoon of fresh elderflowers and 1 tablespoon
of fresh chamomile flowers. Cover with $1\,^1/_2$ mugs of cold
water and bring to the boil, simmering for 10 minutes.
Leave until pleasantly warm and then bathe the eyes in
the usual way.

Rose Petal Lotion

ROSES DON'T simply smell and look good – they can do you good too. They are part of the herbalist's traditional pharmacopoeia and are valued for their anti-inflammatory, cleansing and anti-depressant properties. Try this rose petal lotion for sore eyes and see how effective this flower can be.

Shred 4 red rose petals into 1 cup of cold water, discarding the lower part of the petals, bring to the boil and simmer for 10 minutes. Leave to cool, then apply as a cold compress, on cotton wool pads.

Salt Water

THIS IS a traditional remedy for sore eyes.

Add 1 level teaspoon of sea salt to $\frac{1}{2}$ pint (275 ml) of cold water. Bring to the boil and stir until the salt dissolves. Cool before using.

Quick Tips

Eat plenty of *carrots*, which contain vitamin A – essential to night sight.

Fresh *cucumber slices* placed on the eyelids will help to soothe tired eyes.

Apply a cotton wool compress soaked in *cold tea* to the eyes.

Apply the warm flesh of a *baked apple* to the eyelids.

Pads dipped in refrigerated *witch hazel* are refreshingly astringent.

Warm *chamomile tea bags* on the eyelids can help relieve inflammation.

Slices of *raw potato* soothe puffy eyes.

Rub a stye with a *gold wedding ring* to encourage it to disappear.

CHAPTER SIX

Digestion

*D*id you know that when you serve sage with pork or mint with lamb, you're following traditional medicine? Everyday herbs were traditionally used to help the digestion cope with rich meats like these. Should prevention fail, the kitchen garden also provides standbys to relieve indigestion, often just as effective as those offered by modern medicine. Many — such as oil of peppermint, recommended by doctors today to counteract spasms — have been used for hundreds of years. Here are some garden remedies and storecupboard buys to help.

Ginger

GINGER 'IS of an heating and digesting qualitie, and is profitable for the stomacke', said the physician John Gerard in 1597. Nowadays it is particularly recommended for nausea, including morning sickness and travel sickness – even astronauts have taken ginger into space. Take pieces of crystallized ginger to nibble during journeys, try ginger tea (one teaspoon of grated ginger infused in a cup of freshly boiled water for 10 minutes), or make your own ginger ale.

Soften a large piece of fresh ginger root with a rolling pin to help release the oil. Add to 1 pint (550 ml) of boiling water and simmer for 20 minutes. Strain, add honey to taste, and top up with sparkling mineral water.

Note – too much ginger can cause indigestion if you're sensitive to it, so sip with care.

Chamomile Tea

CHAMOMILE HAS been called the 'mother of the gut' for its soothing properties; it also relieves insomnia and stress. If you have a tendency to indigestion, or simply don't want to be kept awake by drinking coffee at night, try a cup of this delicate tea after meals.

Take 10 fresh chamomile flowers or 1 teaspoon of dried and infuse in a mug of freshly boiled water for 10 minutes. Strain and drink 3 times each day. In summer, chill the tea and blend with pineapple juice, which contains enzymes that help the digestion.

Lemon Barley Water

LEMON BARLEY water is a delicious kitchen remedy for diarrhoea. It helps replace lost fluids.

Cover 4 oz (125 g) of pearl barley with water and bring to the boil. Strain, return the barley to the pan and add 1 $^1\!/_2$ pints (825 ml) of water and the grated rind of 1 lemon. Simmer until the barley is cooked, topping up with water as required, and strain. Sweeten as required and leave to cool.

Marshmallow Tincture

MARSHMALLOW HAS a healing effect on all mucous membranes, so it can help sore mouths as well as stomachs. More than simply soothing, it's also said to combat the inflammation present if you have an ulcer or colitis. You can grow marshmallow in your garden, or obtain it dried from herbalists. It makes one of the most pleasant-tasting of herbal teas – prepare as for chamomile tea, above, but if you need to, sweeten it with a little honey. Alternatively, if you're prepared to sacrifice a small bottle of spirits, you can make the following tincture, which should keep for a year.

Put $1\frac{1}{2}$ oz (40 g) of dried marshmallow flowers or twice that amount of fresh into a screw-top jar and cover with $\frac{1}{2}$ pint (275 ml) of spirits. Seal the jar and store in a dark place for a fortnight. (Shake the jar from time to time.) Then strain the liquid through muslin and throw away the herbs. Take 1 teaspoon, 3 times a day after meals, in $\frac{1}{2}$ cup of freshly boiled water, which reduces the alcohol content – important for sensitive stomachs.

Peppermint Tea

PEPPERMINT IS the indigestion remedy that everybody knows, and it is easy to grow your own mint. Take it as tea after meals (black peppermint is best) or, to help colic or irritable bowel, mix one drop of oil of peppermint in a teaspoon of vodka, then dissolve it in hot water. Like tea, oil of peppermint contains tannin and it has a strong, fast-acting effect on the digestive system. For this reason it is best to alternate peppermint tea with soothers such as chamomile. Avoid it if you have heartburn, which it can provoke rather than cure.

To make peppermint tea, add 1 scant teaspoon of dried mint or 1 heaped teaspoon of fresh to a mug of freshly boiled water. Leave for 10 minutes, then strain and drink.

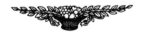

Gruel

GRUEL IS a thin porridge used for centuries to
tempt invalids' appetites. Made from slippery
elm bark, available from herbalists and pharmacists,
it soothes the digestive tract; made with arrowroot,
it will curb diarrhoea.

Mix 1 tablespoon of powdered slippery elm bark or
arrowroot to a paste with a little milk or water. Top up
with hot milk or water, stirring all the time, and flavour
with a cinnamon stick, or add to cooked porridge oats if
you want a more substantial dish.

Garlic

GARLIC IS an ancient cure-all that's rapidly gaining
scientific respect. Medical researchers have found that it
can help prevent heart disease and fight infection – and
that goes not just for colds but for food poisoning too.
Our grandmothers knew this all along, but now
researchers have studied the way garlic can eliminate

harmful bacteria in the gut or restore the balance
after a course of antibiotics: two cloves a day are
recommended. Mixed with milk, garlic can also
be a cure for constipation.

Pour 1 cup of cold milk into a small pan, add 5 peeled
cloves of garlic and boil until the garlic has softened.
Remove the garlic and drink just before you go to sleep.

❖

Yoghurt and Rice

YOGHURT AND rice can settle an acid stomach. The
traditional recipe uses curds, but plain, preferably live,
yoghurt will do very well in its place. Live yoghurt
contains the bacteria bifidus and acidophilus, which
help maintain a healthy balance in the gut.

Soak a handful of cooked rice in a glass of cold water
overnight. Next morning, strain, mix with a carton of
plain yoghurt and eat for breakfast.

Caraway, Cardamom and Cinnamon

THE THREE Cs – caraway, cardamom and cinnamon – are spices that warm your insides. They have what's called a carminative action, which means they can relieve colic and bloating.

Caraway – infuse 1 teaspoon of seeds in a mug of hot water for 10 minutes. Strain, and drink before meals.
Cardamom – crush 6 cardamom pods to release the oil then cover with $^1/_2$ pint (275 ml) of hot water. Infuse for 10 minutes, then strain.
Cinnamon – flavour hot milk with a cinnamon stick or $^1/_2$ teaspoon of ground cinnamon.

Fennel

FENNEL HAS a refreshingly tangy taste and was once 'much used for those that are grown fat', as one 17th-century writer put it; it's also thought to encourage a plentiful supply of breast milk. It grows vigorously in the garden, producing quantities of seed heads. Try this fennel tea to relieve flatulence.

Pound 1 1/2 oz (40 g) of fennel seeds and cover with 1 pint (550 ml) of freshly boiled water. Leave to stand for 10 minutes, strain, and drink 3 times a day, after meals.

❖

Aromatherapy Massage

AN AROMATHERAPY massage does more than 'rub it better', though many doctors believe touch helps close the nerves' gateway to pain. Using essential oils will help you benefit from the healing power of plants even if you can't face the thought of food or drink.

Mix 2 drops of essential oil of geranium to tone, 2 drops of lavender for pain relief, and 2 drops of peppermint, known to help indigestion, in 1 tablespoon of warmed almond oil. Massage gently into the abdomen using circular strokes in a clockwise direction and then cover the abdomen with a warm, damp towel. (Replace with another before it cools.)

Mrs Russell's Oaten Jelly

THIS IS an old family recipe, says one *Good Housekeeping* reader. It's a soothing dish for anyone recovering from a bout of gastric trouble and is an excellent way of tempting poor appetites. Oat flour is available from specialist healthfood suppliers.

Blend $2^1/_2$ oz (65 g) of oat flour with a little water taken from 1 pint (550 ml). Boil the rest of the water and slowly pour on to the blended flour, stirring until thick. Return to the pan and add $^1/_2$ oz (15 g) of butter or polyunsaturated margarine. Bring to the boil and simmer for 7 minutes, stirring all the time, until it thickens. Add sugar or honey to taste and serve as a pudding, with milk or thin cream.

❖

Potato Juice

POTATO JUICE is a traditional way to relieve stomach cramps and, it's said, even ulcers. Avoid green potatoes, which can be poisonous. Alternatives include cabbage juice and, an old cottage standby, the water new potatoes have been boiled in.

Peel and scrub ¹/₂ lb (250 g) of potatoes, then chop into bite-sized pieces before liquidizing or putting in a food processor. Add lemon juice to taste. Take 2 tablespoons before each meal. Do not take for longer than 24 hours.

Figs

SYRUP OF figs is a well-known cure for constipation. Today most experts prefer fibre as a natural remedy, but if you're desperate try the following recipe.

Soak 2 oz (50 g) of dried figs and 2 oz (50 g) of prunes in 1 pint (550 ml) of water for 8 hours, then bring to the boil and simmer until the fruit is soft and any excess liquid has been reduced. Stir in 1 tablespoon of treacle, then cool and blend in a food processor. Pour into a jam jar and keep in the fridge. Take 1 dessertspoonful as needed.

Quick Tips

One drop of *oil of cloves* taken in a teaspoon of sugar can relieve nausea.

Stewed rhubarb helps relieve constipation.

Juniper berries or a splash of gin in hot water may settle your stomach.

Dry white toast helps treat diarrhoea.

Soaked linseed adds bulk – the approved way to cope with constipation.

Chickweed can relieve constipation – serve in salad.

Senna pods are a classic laxative, but should not be taken regularly.

Take half a teaspoon of *bicarbonate of soda* in water for flatulence.

Eat *grated apple* to treat sudden diarrhoea.

Sniff *pepper* to cure hiccoughs.

CHAPTER SEVEN

Stress

*I*s stress a 20th-century complaint? Not at all: imagine the pressures of living when poverty was rife and infant mortality high. Country people had their own ways of coping with it. In Lark Rise to Candleford, *Flora Thompson describes how the household drank chamomile tea 'to soothe the nerves and as a general tonic'.*

Stress is not always harmful, but excessive stress can impair immunity. If that's the state you're approaching, set aside at least 15 minutes a day to do nothing but relax, and try these gentle remedies. Do make sure to see your doctor, though, if stress continues to affect your health.

Cumin

CUMIN IS an Oriental spice that helps counter anxiety.
Try it as an infusion or a tea.

Pound 1 teaspoon of cumin seeds and add to 1 mug of
boiled water. Leave for 10 minutes, then strain and drink.

Valerian

VALERIAN IS one of the strongest sedatives in the
plant world. It's said to be the herb the Pied
Piper used to tempt the rats out of Hamelin,
and certainly it was in general use as a tranquillizer
until the end of the Second World War. Because it's so
powerful valerian is usually combined with other herbs;
it can also be bought in tablet form.

Mix $^1/_2$ oz (15 g) of dried valerian root with 1 oz (25 g)
of fresh mint leaves. Pour over 1 pint (550 ml) of boiled
water and leave for several hours before straining. Drink
warm or cold, no more than 3 times a day.

Vervain Tea

VERVAIN (VERBENA) has been valued for its
stress-relieving properties since Roman times –
indeed, it is so effective that it was once associated
with witchcraft. It has a bitter taste so sweeten this tea
with a spoonful of honey.

Take 1 scant teaspoon of dried vervain or 1 heaped teaspoon
of fresh vervain leaves and flowers and cover with 1 mug
of freshly boiled water. Leave to stand for 10 minutes,
then strain and serve. Add honey to taste, if you like.

❖

Basil and Sage

THESE HERBS can help you absorb the emotional shock
caused by good or bad news. (Physical shock resulting
from injury is quite different, and in this case nothing
should be given by mouth at all.)

Using equal parts of basil and sage, put 1 scant teaspoon
of dried herbs or 1 heaped teaspoon of fresh into a jug and
cover with $1/2$ pint (275 ml) of boiling water. Leave to
stand for 10 minutes, then strain and drink.

Massage

ANYONE WHO has been to a health farm knows
that a fragrant massage makes you feel languorous
and completely relaxed. Massage is an Eastern
and a European tradition but one that stiff-
necked Northerners could do well to adopt.
Here's what to do.

To benefit fully, you'll need to use the pure essential oils
recommended for aromatherapy. Put 4 teaspoons of
warmed almond oil in a cup and blend with 3 drops each
of calming and anti-depressant rose and geranium
essential oils, plus sandalwood or neroli to intensify the
effect. Ask your partner to rub the oil into his or her palms
and, using the whole of the hand, to make long, firm
strokes either side of your spine towards your neck and
then down your sides. Kneading movements can be used
on your bottom and thighs; long, sliding ones from your
toes and fingers along your limbs; light circular
movements over your neck and, in a clockwise direction,
over the belly; soft strokes over the face. Avoid massaging
the throat or over varicose veins. Finish by relaxing,
wrapped in a warm towel, with your eyes closed.

Quick Tips

A few drops of *rosemary oil* in the bath will stimulate and refresh.

Add two *cloves* to a cup of herbal tea to help lift depression.

Porridge may relieve depression: oats are full of vitamin B, which is vital to the nervous system.

Chop *fresh basil* in salads or add to sauces. It stimulates the mind as well as the taste buds.

Try *thyme* to relieve anxiety.

In folk medicine, *walnuts* were believed to help the nervous system because they resemble the brain. They may also lower cholesterol.

CHAPTER EIGHT

Insomnia

*I*f a good night's sleep is something you can only dream of, try one of these remedies based on traditional herbal medicine. Many plants are natural sedatives and make pleasant herbal teas, well worth substituting for caffeine-based drinks and alcohol, which can add to sleep problems.

To maximize your chances of getting off to sleep easily, avoid heavy meals in the evening. A soothing bath followed by a sedative herbal tea last thing at night should put you in the right frame of mind for sleep, but if you still have problems relaxing, try some of the remedies for stress (pages 65–9), too.

Sleep Pillow

A SLEEP pillow tucked under your usual one can waft
you off to sleep.

Make up a small square of cotton lawn and fill with a
generous handful of dried hops, plus a scattering of
fragrant herbs. Dried lavender and lemon balm or rose
petals and mint are two sweetly scented combinations.

❖

Herbal Bath

A DEEP herbal bath is a wonderful preparation for sleep.
Drink a cup of one of the sedative herbal teas –
chamomile, lime flower or lemon balm – as well, and
make sure everything is prepared so you can go straight
to bed afterwards. You'll barely be able to keep your
eyes open.

Add 2 drops each of essential oils of chamomile and
sandalwood to the bath water while it is running – it
should be pleasantly warm. Place cotton wool soaked in
chamomile tea over your eyes and lie in the bath for 5 to
10 minutes. Then go straight to bed.

Chamomile, Lemon Balm and Lime Flower Tea

THIS TEA combines three soothing herbs in a calming
bedtime drink. As with all herbal teas, the amount taken
is very much a matter of taste. Fresh ingredients are
better but are less concentrated than dried herbs, so you
need to use more – but not so much that the result is
unpalatable. On the other hand, it's a mistake to drink
large quantities of dilute liquid before bedtime.
Experiment to find the right mixture for you.

Mix equal parts of chamomile flowers, lemon balm leaves
and lime (linden) flowers. Using 1 scant teaspoon of dried
herbs or 1 heaped teaspoon of fresh, add to 1 large teacup
of freshly boiled water and leave to stand for 10 minutes.
Strain before drinking.

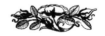

Quick Tips

Starchy foods such as *banana, bread or biscuits*, taken in moderation before bedtime, encourage sleep.

Take a teaspoon of *honey in chamomile tea*.

Put two drops of *chamomile oil* on your pillow.

A drink of warm fresh *orange juice*, sweetened with honey, will help induce sleep.

Put sprigs of *dill* on your pillow.

Lettuce is a natural sedative, so eat plenty in salads or try lettuce soup.

CHAPTER NINE

Circulation

*C*old hands may mean a warm heart but they may also indicate poor circulation, and that can be bad for your health. Because the blood carries nutrients and oxygen round the body and takes away waste, it's important for healthy tissues. Exercise is one of the best ways to get it moving, so try making time for a brisk walk every day, but you could also try to stimulate the blood flow in other ways. The remedies in this chapter can help to relieve conditions as varied as varicose veins, cramp and chilblains — all of which are caused by sluggish circulation.

Hawthorn Tonic

HAWTHORN BERRIES are valued for heart complaints and high blood pressure, because they have a gentle strengthening effect on the heart. It goes without saying that anyone who's worried about heart problems should seek medical advice, but if your doctor agrees, try a refreshing hawthorn tonic.

Crush 3 teaspoons of berries and infuse in a large mug of hot water for 15 minutes. Strain, then drink, adding a pinch of cinnamon to taste, if you like. You can also use hawthorn berries like redcurrants, to make jelly.

Ginger Foot Powder

THIS HELPS prevent chilblains. Boots and thick socks are recommended for chilblain sufferers, but foot powder will help keep your feet warm if you want to wear light shoes or like to walk round in slippers.

Mix 1 teaspoon of powdered ginger with a handful of cornflour or talcum powder. Dust it inside your shoes.

Garlic

GARLIC IS good for you, as people have known for thousands of years. Now it's official: clinical trials have shown that garlic has a beneficial effect on blood cholesterol, and the secret is thought to lie in the compound allicin, which gives garlic its taste – and smell.

Try mashing cloves of garlic into salad, grating them over vegetables, extracting the juice to take neat or in salad dressing, or chewing them raw. Finish by chewing plenty of parsley to sweeten the breath.

Nettles

NETTLES ARE a folk remedy well-known for their beneficial effect on the heart and circulation, and as they are a good source of iron they help combat anaemia too. Young nettle leaves are delicious steamed, like spinach, or served in a salad. You could also try:

Nettle tea. Take 2 oz (50 g) of fresh nettle leaves or 1 oz (25 g) of dried and boil for 3 minutes in 1 pint (550 ml) of water. Leave for 10 minutes, then strain and drink 1 cup, 3 times a day.

Nettle soup. Soften 1 finely chopped onion and 2 crushed cloves of garlic in a little vegetable oil over a low heat. Add sufficient flour to make a paste and gradually add 1 pint (550 ml) of light stock. Stir until it thickens then add 1 lb (500 g) of washed young nettle leaves; cover and simmer. When the nettles are cooked, take the mixture off the hob and cool for a few minutes. Blend in a food processor or liquidizer and then reheat, adding milk and seasoning to taste.

Cayenne Sling

CAYENNE, OR chilli powder, gives the circulation
a boost. It's often used in commercial heat sprays
and rubs because it brings the blood to surface.
Taken internally, it's thought to prevent blood
clotting. In the P.G. Wodehouse novels, Jeeves
laced raw egg and milk with cayenne and used
it as a hangover cure for Bertie Wooster. Raw
egg is no longer recommended because of the
risk of salmonella, but why not try the following?
It will certainly give you a boost, and it may
even cure a hangover.

Add 1 carton of plain yoghurt, a few drops of
Worcestershire sauce and $^1/_2$ teaspoon of cayenne pepper
to 1 cup of cold milk. Whisk together and drink.

Quick Tips

Roast onion helps heal chilblains – simply press it on the affected area.

A mustard footbath warms cold feet – and can help headaches and colds too.

Salt tablets are good for cramp (take only if your blood pressure is normal).

Cider vinegar can be applied morning and night to shrink varicose veins.

Soak a handful of fresh *pot marigold heads in distilled witch hazel* for half an hour then apply the flowers to varicose veins (don't use on broken skin).

Horse chestnut essence in a footbath improves circulation and soothes chilblains.

CHAPTER TEN

Just for Women

Traditionally, women have been the key to the family's health, dispensing advice and medicine in equal proportions. So it's not surprising that there are many folk remedies specifically for women's health, designed to sort out blips in the menstrual cycle, help with nursing and childbirth, and smooth the passage of the menopause. Modern medicine is rediscovering the value of many of these plant-based treatments, but there's no need to buy expensive patent medicines because many remedies can easily be made at home.

Cranberry Juice

THIS TRADITIONAL remedy for cystitis is now backed up by modern medicine because, as generations of women know, it works! You can buy cranberry juice in supermarkets, but to reap the full benefit, make your own from fresh or frozen berries.

Press $1/2$ lb (250 g) of cranberries through a sieve or put them in a food processor until finely mashed. Add a little water if the consistency is too thick. Stir, and drink a glassful 3 times a day until the condition clears. In between, flush your system by drinking plenty of plain water. Avoid citrus juices, tea and coffee.

❖

Marigold Tea

MARIGOLD TEA can help you cope with the flushes and hormonal swings of the menopause.

Put 1 scant teaspoon of dried marigold heads or 1 heaped teaspoon of fresh flowers into a jug and pour over 1 mug of freshly boiled water. Cover and leave to stand for 10 minutes, then strain. Drink several times a day.

Marshmallow

MARSHMALLOW CAN soothe all ailments of the
mucous membranes, whether in the digestive or
reproductive tract. If you suffer from cystitis,
try this gentle remedy, which can be used as a
wash or taken by mouth, as a tea.

Place 1 oz (25 g) of marshmallow root (available from
herbalists) in a saucepan. Cover with $^3/_4$ pint (415 ml) of
cold water and bring to the boil. Simmer for 1 hour, then
strain, first through a sieve and then through coffee filter
paper.

❖

Mrs Thomas's Beetroot Tonic

THIS PICK-ME-UP has been used by women in
Mrs Thomas's family for generations. 'The recipe
was given to me by my grandmother,' explains
Mrs Thomas. Beetroot is traditionally thought
to be good for the nervous system, and it helps
prevent fatigue and dizziness.

Wash 3 lb (1½ kg) of fresh raw beetroot and slice, unpeeled, into a large bowl. Cover with 2 lb (1 kg) of brown sugar and leave to stand for 3 days, stirring from time to time. Strain through muslin into a clean jug and add 1 bottle of Guinness or stout. Stir well, bottle, and seal before storing (not too tightly or pressure will build up). Drink 1 small sherry glass a day.

Raspberry Leaf Tea

PAINFUL PERIODS? Relief in labour? Try raspberry leaf tea, an old country cure-all for menstrual cramps which is reputed to help labour pains too. If you want to see if it can help in childbirth, drink three cups a day *during the last three months of pregancy only*. Because the tea is a uterine stimulant, it's important not to drink it earlier.

Take 2 oz (50 g) of fresh young raspberry leaves or 1 oz (25 g) of dried and pour over 1 scant pint (500 ml) of freshly boiled water. Leave to stand for 15 minutes, then strain before drinking.

PMS Salad

THIS SALAD uses knowledge culled from the past to deal with a modern problem. Over 70 per cent of women are thought to suffer from premenstrual syndrome, with its symptoms of bloating, breast pain, headache and irritability. This salad combines ingredients that are rich in vitamins and have a mild diuretic effect to combat water retention.

Mix together a selection of the following salad vegetables: lettuce leaves (sedative), dandelion leaves and chopped celery (mildly diuretic), parsley, young nettle tops, spinach and watercress (good sources of vitamins and minerals, including iron). Toss in a salad dressing made from walnut oil (thought to help with period problems), lemon juice and a little crushed garlic. Eat daily, as a side salad, in sandwiches, or with fish, meat or eggs as a main course.

Rosewater and Lady's Mantle Wash

LADY'S MANTLE has been used for four centuries for 'wounds inwards and outwards'. It can relieve what is delicately called 'feminine itching'.

Soak a handful of lady's mantle in 1 cup of rosewater (available from pharmacies or herbalists) overnight. Strain twice through coffee filter paper and bathe the skin gently, twice a day.

❖

Lovage Tea

LOVAGE TEA can help relieve the uncomfortable premenstrual bloating that many women experience. Lovage is wild celery and grows like wildfire in the garden, so you may like to confine it by growing it in a bucket buried in the earth, as recommended for mint.

Take 1 heaped teaspoon of chopped fresh lovage and cover with 1 mug of freshly boiled water. Leave for 10 minutes, then strain and add honey if required. (Lovage is bitter and can be an acquired taste.) Stir, and drink 3 times a day.

Quick Tips

Tie *six corks* in an old stocking and keep them in the bed – an old wives' solution to night cramps.

Massage *coconut oil* into your skin during pregnancy to help prevent stretch marks.

Dissolve half a teaspoon of *bicarbonate of soda* in a glass of water and drink to relieve acidity, and hence cystitis.

Eat *starchy snacks* (crispbread, nuts or seeds) every three hours for PMS.

Try *sorrel tea* to relieve PMS.

Put a few drops of *tea tree oil* on a tampon if you suffer from thrush.

Take *fennel or caraway tea* for period pains.

Witch hazel applied on a compress soothes cystitis.

Use *cold marigold tea* as a vaginal wash.

Eat *fennel* to increase milk production.

CHAPTER ELEVEN

Remedies for Children

Many mothers turn to traditional medicine when their children are ill because there's something very comforting about using remedies that have been handed down through the generations. If your mother used homemade gripe water to settle a sore stomach, or made you an inhalation to shift a stubborn cough, you'll remember how gentle and effective they were. They should only be used for mild conditions and, unless otherwise stated, reserved for children over one year old. Any small child who has diarrhoea, pain or fever for more than 24 hours should see a doctor. If you're worried for any reason, don't hesitate to call the GP.

Dill Water

THIS IS a traditional remedy for three-month colic, which makes babies fretful in the evening just when you most want them to sleep. Explanations that have been put forward for the condition include allergy, tension and an immature digestive system. You can take measures to combat all three by eliminating onions, spicy foods and too much fruit from your diet if you are breast-feeding, wrapping your baby in a light shawl and rocking gently while you both relax, and trying the following colic drops.

Put 1 teaspoon of dill seeds in a cup and top up with freshly boiled water. Leave for 20 minutes then strain through a coffee filter paper. Give 1 teaspoon of the dill water before each feed, but before your baby is really hungry and will reject everything but milk. Fennel seeds can be used in the same way.

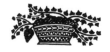

Rose Hip Tonic

ROSE HIP tonic contains all the goodness of vitamin C-rich rose hips without the tooth-rotting qualities of the original syrup.

Take 1 teaspoon of dried rose hips or $1\frac{1}{2}$ teaspoons of fresh and mix with a pinch of ground cinnamon. Pour over 1 cup of freshly boiled water and leave to stand for 10 minutes before straining. Add a squeeze of lemon juice and, if needed, a little honey to sweeten. Drink as a tea.

❖

Rice-angee for Tummy Upsets

THIS POPULAR Indian treatment for diarrhoea has been known since the time of the Raj. Always seek medical advice for babies and young toddlers with acute diarrhoea because they quickly become dehydrated – the usual treatment is oral rehydration salts. Once they're on the mend, you can try weaning them back to health with this recipe, which adds salt and sugar to restore the minerals and energy lost.

It should be made fresh every day, comments
Lakshmi Aima, whose recipe this is.

Put 1 1/2 pints (825 ml) of cold water and a handful of
ground rice in a saucepan, bring to the boil and leave to
cool. Stir in 1 level teaspoon of salt, and taste – 'It should
not taste more salty than tears,' says Lakshmi. Mix in 8 level
teaspoons of sugar and give to children 1/2 cup at a time.

❖

Baby Massage

BABY MASSAGE is part of everyday baby care in the
Far East. Soothing oils such as chamomile can
help relieve tension and colic.

Warm an eggcupful of almond oil by standing it in a bowl
of warm water. Add 1 drop of chamomile oil and mix well.
Lay your baby on a warm towel on your lap for the
massage. Be guided by your baby's reactions, but as a
general rule, use light, soothing strokes, working from the
fingers and toes along the limbs towards the heart. Use
light, circular strokes over the tummy, then turn your
baby over and work up either side of the spine and down
the back. Finish by wrapping your baby in a warm towel.

Alternative First Aid

Some remedies have never disappeared but have been produced commercially for years. You'll find most of the following in pharmacies, though you may have to ask for them or be prepared to search the back shelves. Stock your own alternative first-aid kit with them and use to treat wounds, bites and stings.

Arnica cream – a balm for bruises and sprains. Keep away from open wounds because it can irritate.
Calendula (marigold) cream – a soothing skin treatment for cuts and grazes.
Comfrey ointment – stimulates wound healing.
Distilled witch hazel – astringent and cooling.
Lavender oil – a natural antiseptic. Buy the pure essential oil aromatherapists recommend and use it neat for bites and stings.
Tea tree oil – a traditional Australian cure-all, tea tree oil is antiseptic and antifungal. Use it for scratches, cuts and sores.

Remedies can be used in combination. For example, where skin is bruised but not broken, treat with astringent witch hazel, followed by soothing arnica cream.

Glossary

Because it's important to use the right plant when you try your hand at traditional medicine, look for the Latin rather than the popular name when you buy. The word *officinalis* means that it has medical properties.

basil (*Ocimum basilicum*)
betony – see wood betony
bladderwrack (*Fucus vesiculosus*)
chamomile (*Chamomilla recutita*)
cowslip (*Primula veris*)
dill (*Anethum graveolens*)
elder (*Sambucus nigra*)
eyebright (*Euphrasia officinalis*)
fennel (*Foeniculum officinale*)
feverfew (*Tanacetum parthenium*)
geranium (*Perlargonium odorantissimum*)
ginger (*Zingiber officinale*)
golden seal (*Hydrastis canadensis*)
hawthorn (*Crataegus oxyacantha*)
lady's mantle (*Alchemilla vulgaris*)

lavender (*Lavandula augustifolia*)
lemon balm (*Melissa officinalis*)
liquorice (*Glycyrrhiza glabra*)
lovage (*Levisticum officinale*)
marigold (*Calendula officinalis*)
marjoram (*Origanum vulgare*)
marshmallow (*Althaea officinalis*)
meadowsweet (*Filipendula ulmaria*)
mugwort (*Artemisia vulgaris*)
passionflower (*Passiflora incarnata*)
peppermint (*Mentha piperita*)
raspberry (*Rubus idaeus*)
red sage (*Salvia officinalis*)
rosemary (*Rosmarinus officinalis*)
rue (*Ruta graveolens*)
slippery elm (*Ulmus fulva*)
thyme (*Thymus vulgaris*)
valerian (*Valeriana officinalis*)
vervain (*Verbena officinalis*)
white willow (*Salix alba*)
wood betony (*Betonica officinalis*; *Stachys officinalis*)

List of Suppliers and Useful Addresses

G. Baldwin & Co, 171/173 Walworth Road, London, SE17 1RW(020 7703 5550)
    sales@baldwins.co.uk – mail order.
Barwinnock Herbs, Barrhill, Ayrshire, KA26 0RB (01465 821338)
    herbs@barwinnock.com – mail order.
Culpeper Ltd, Hadstock Road, Linton, Cambridge, CB1 6NJ (01223 891196)
    www.culpeper.co.uk – mail order and Birmingham branch.
The Herb Farm, Peppard Road, Reading, RG4 9NJ (01189 724220)
    www.herbfarm.co.uk – mail order and Reading branch.
Neal's Yard Remedies, Peacemarsh, Gillingham, Dorset, SP8 4EU (01747
    834600) mail@nealsyardremedies.com – mail order and various
    branches.
Shirley Price Aromatherapy Ltd, Essentia House, Upper Bond Street, Hinckley,
    LE10 1RS (01455 615466) www.shirleyprice.com – aromatherapy
    supplies by mail order.
Tisserand Aromatherapy Institute, 65 Church Road, Hove, Sussex, BN3 7BA
    (01273 325666) - aromatherapy supplies by mail order.

For individual advice on herbal medicine, you can consult a medical herbalist. To
find one, contact the National Institute of Medical Herbalists, Elm House,
54 Mary Arches Street, Exeter, EX4 3BA (01392 426022)
nimh@ukexeter.freeserve.co.uk

Index